Managing Fibromyalgia

Getting to know your aggravators

Managing Fibromyalgia
Subtitle: Getting to know your Aggravators

Copyright © 2008 Pati Chandler
All rights reserved.

Cover design:
Copyright © 2008 Lee Emory
All rights reserved.

Treble Heart Books
1284 Overlook Dr.
Sierra Vista, AZ 85635-5512
http://www.trebleheartbooks.com

Edited by Lee Emory, 2008

Library of Congress Control Number: 2008904486

Tradesize paperback ISBN: 978-1-932695-71-7
Case bound hard back ISBN: 978-1-932695-72-4

Table of Contents

Acknowledgement

I want to thank Arlene Van Belle, fellow author, best friend, and chief cheerleader, who has been with me from day one, for her never-ending encouragement and upliftment. It was her light that has guided me onto this path and I am eternally grateful.

Thank you to Anita Cibelli, my friend and travel companion, who has stood behind me, gently nudging and encouraging me all the way.

Thank you to Artie Estridge, my new friend and soon to be Ph.D., for her words of encouragement in this endeavor, while we both learned along the way.

Thank you to Jane Oelke, N.D., Ph.D. for permission to use her artwork and for her kind words.

And of course, I heartily thank K. Bhatt, D.O., of Mishawaka for his accurate diagnosis so that I would know where to begin.

I especially want to thank Lee Emory, my publisher, for taking a chance on me and for her editorial assistance in bringing this book out to where it is needed.

Dedication

I dedicate this book to every person who has Fibromyalgia, but most especially to every person who has subjected herself or himself to the rheumatologists who are doing the tests and studies to benefit us. I thank you all.

Managing Fibromyalgia

—*Getting to know your Aggravators*

by

Pati Chandler

Published in the U.S.A.

Treble Heart Books
1284 Overlook Dr.
Sierra Vista, AZ 85635

http://www.trebleheartbooks.com

PART I

About Fibromyalgia

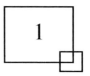

1

Fibromyalgia

The word itself conjures up a multitude of feelings in the more than six million Americans who have Fibromyalgia.[1] To those who don't have it the word only brings a "what's that?" query. It is a rather new word to the English language, having been coined only about two decades ago. When broken down into its three parts, *fibro*, Latin for fibrous tissue, *myo*, Greek for muscle, and *algia*, Latin for pain, it is fairly self-explanatory. Simple.

Not so the explaination of the condition or syndrome. Because a syndrome, by definition, is a collection of symptoms, this is the most accurate term and so the condition is often called Fibromyalgia Syndrome or FMS.

Fibromyalgia is considered a rheumatic condition, which, according to the National Institute of Health, means that it's a medical condition that impairs the joints and soft tissues and causes chronic pain.[2]

There is no one treatment or combination of treatments for all Fibromyalgia sufferers. Each person's Fibromyalgia manifests somewhat differently, making it hard for the physician to treat. And though the symptoms are many and varied, they intertwine to "make up" the syndrome, with pain and fatigue the common denominator.[3]

Symptoms

What are the symptoms? "Practically everything known to man," would be the answer given by a person with Fibromyalgia. But pain is the symptom that tops the list and pretty much defines the entire subject. Muscular pain. Joint pain. Neck pain. Headache pain. Jaw and facial pain. Lower back pain. Upper arm pain. Wrist pain. Hip pain. Leg pain. Foot pain. In other words, think…a severe case of the flu where everything hurts, the muscles and joints in the body don't work properly and utter exhaustion rules the day.[4]

With a major flare-up, this pain *in all those places* is severe and sharp. When the flare-up subsides, the pain is still there—it virtually never goes away because it is a chronic malady. This pain, however, is now in the form of constant and relentless aches all over. This pain is not so totally debilitating as the more extreme flare-up, but in its own way, being so unmercifully persistent and so constant, it's no wonder depression is a common symptom.[5]

It simply wears a body down. The Colorado River carving the Grand Canyon deeper and deeper comes to mind.

Pain is only the first symptom. The full list of symptoms is legion. An individual may not have all the symptoms, but it is very common to have most of them. They include, but are not limited to, an all-consuming fatigue, numbness or tingling sensations in the hands and feet, sudden momentary electric-shock-like sensations in the hands and feet,[6] irritable bowel syndrome, restless leg syndrome, dizziness, and lowered resistance to infection. Chemical sensitivity, inhaled or ingested.[7] Odors, food additives or even some medications can initiate either allergy symptoms like burning eyes and throat with runny nose or body symptoms of nausea, headache, dizziness, vomiting and body pain.

There is a heightened sensitivity to touch, cold, heat, odors, noise and bright lights, in addition to memory difficulties and confusion (sometimes called fibro fog), anxiety or panic attacks, abdominal pain with bloating and/or nausea, and moodiness.[8]

Some symptoms actually mimic other conditions such as chronic fatigue syndrome, carpal tunnel syndrome, arthritis, even lupus, muscular sclerosis and Alzheimer's.[9]

The most common symptom for all people with Fibromyalgia is a total lack of deep, restful, restorative, Stage 4 sleep. This is the period of sleep where the body repairs and replenishes itself, healing the multitudinous tiny tears in muscle tissue we all get during the day,[10] and when our body brings in oxygen to those areas that have become depleted during the day. During every eight-hour night of sleep, those with FMS are constantly interrupted by "bursts of awakened brain activity similar to wakefulness,"[8] prohibiting the Stage 4 sleep.

In other words, there is a malfunction at the most basic level, the level at which the body should be healing itself.[11] For those without FMS, it would be akin to just drifting off to sleep, then jerking awake, constantly, all night long...*every* night.

It's no wonder FMS sufferers wake up feeling like they have

been dragged a mile down a railroad track. And they wake exhausted. Some sufferers have reported that getting out of bed in the morning involved crawling on hands and knees just to get to the bathroom. All-over body pain upon waking is a symptom all FMS sufferers endure.[12]

The painful muscles are weak and don't move properly. The aching legs and ankles feel like lead weights are attached to them and walking becomes a not-so-simple task. *Holding a cup of coffee must be done with two hands due to weak arms and wrists or tingly and numb hands and fingers.*

The memory difficulties and confusion that are so prevalent with Fibromyalgia sufferers are no less imposing. The mind tends to wander in the middle of what you are saying or doing. If driving, for example, forgetting where you are going or even how to get home is a very scary proposition and a panic attack can occur. But then, a panic attack can also occur while standing at the kitchen sink doing the dishes.

Adding insult to injury, another symptom for some is weight gain,[7] which usually adds to depression. Clumsiness and spatial difficulties are not exactly a morale booster either.[13]

With Fibromyalgia every day is different. From day to day the frequency and location of pain and degree of the pain varies—from general body aches to severe and debilitating pain—along with any of the *other* added symptoms that decide to show up.[14]

The Cause

No one knows what causes Fibromyalgia, although researchers have many theories. Some think that the lack of sleep may be a cause, rather than a symptom. Another theory suggests changes in the muscle metabolism caused by decreased blood flow to the muscles may be a cause.[15]

Experts have noted that Fibromyalgia often manifests after an injury or trauma (particularly in the upper spinal region), or following a bacterial or viral infection such as a severe case of bronchitis or the flu. In fact it can manifest following, or along with, any incident that lowers the body's resistance. That is when its fighting forces are at its lowest ebb, which includes emotional trauma or severe stress as well.[16]

Most experts agree that it may be a central nervous system disorder, citing that the nervous system may be supersensitive in some way. Researchers have found elevated levels of a pain-producing nerve chemical, called *Substance P,* in the spinal fluid of FMS sufferers, while at the same time finding too little of the neurotransmitter serotonin, which helps modulate pain perception, mood, sleep, and more.[17] Nevertheless, there is no definitive cause that can be pointed to and declared, "That's what causes it." At least not yet.

2

Diagnosis

Diagnosing Fibromyalgia is a bit of a problem. Fibromyalgia doesn't show up in blood tests or in x-rays. When the FMS sufferer tells his or her doctor the list of symptoms, usually after weeks of feeling all-over pain, weakness and utter exhaustion, the doctor will run a battery of tests to eliminate the usual suspects displaying these and all the rest of the symptoms. The doctor will test for lupus, hypothyroidism, multiple sclerosis, rheumatoid arthritis and so on.[18] All the tests come up negative. Now this should be a good thing. And it is, sort of. At least these serious disorders have been eliminated. The problem lies in the criteria for the diagnosis.

The diagnosis of Fibromyalgia requires only two conditions. The first is that the pain must have been consistent for at least three months. That alone does not sound hopeful. The second condition is that 11 of 18 trigger points should demonstrate pain when slight pressure is applied to these points.[19]

See illustration on next page.

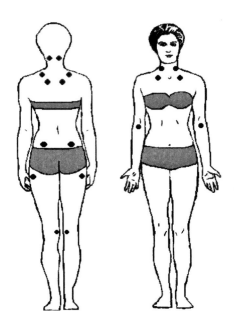

In a non-FMS sufferer there would be no pain at all when these points are pressed. But if Fibromyalgia is the culprit, a slight pressure applied to these points will create a bone-deep, radiating, lasting pain at these sites. This is not an enjoyable procedure. But it is necessary for the proper diagnosis.

There is good news and bad news with a diagnosis of Fibromyalgia. The good news is Fibromyalgia is not progressive or life threatening.[20] The bad news is it is chronic, meaning long-lasting.

Okay. You have a diagnosis, a label. Now what? Knowledge is power. Educate yourself about the syndrome. Google it. Keyword it. Learn all you can through websites such as those listed in Chapter 10, through books, articles and so on. There is information everywhere now and it's updated constantly. Medical testing goes on daily. Individual essays and books such as this are meant for all FMS sufferers in hopes something that helps one may help others. Each FMS sufferer must learn what his or her medical options are, learn what aggravates the symptoms, and learn about self-care…learn what you can do to manage your own health and well-being.

Medical help

Family practitioners are learning more and more about Fibromyalgia, but still your healthcare provider may refer you to a rheumatologist. In 1990 the American College of Rheumatology established the general classification guidelines for this syndrome and they have done much of the research involved in its assessment. In fact rheumatologists Richard H. Gracely, Frank Petzke, Julie M. Wolf and Daniel J. Clauw from the University of Michigan Health System—Chronic Pain and Research Center—actually proved via magnetic resonance imaging (MRI) that Fibromyalgia was a legitimate, painful, medical condition and not an imagined ailment *as had been believed for many years.*[25]

But whether a family doctor or rheumatologist, everyone involved in the care and treatment of Fibromyalgia, as well as those who suffer from the syndrome, agrees the two most important treatments are for restorative, restful sleep and pain relief.[22]

Sleep

Unfortunately, regular sleeping pills haven't proved helpful for FMS sufferers; they don't address Stage 4 sleep. However, there are several prescription medications that help. A low dosage tricyclic antidepressant such as amitriptyline, e.g. Elavil, or a muscle relaxant such as cyclobenzaprine, e.g. Flexeril, has been shown to help get restorative, healing sleep. In addition, a different type of antidepressant called a selective seratonin reuptake inhibitor (SSRI), such as Paxil, has been effective.[23] Some physicians may even recommend an over-the-counter anti-depressant called Sam-e, short for S-adenosylmethionine. In Europe Sam-e is a prescription medication and physicians there have prescribed it for depression, chronic fatigue syndrome and Fibromyalgia for many years.[24]

Be certain your doctor knows ALL the medications, supplements or herbs you are currently taking in order to avoid any negative reactions.

Even though the tricyclic antidepressants and the SSRI's are given to FMS sufferers in a fraction of the dose given for clinical depression, these and all medications are not meant to be used *ad infinatum*. Since Fibromyalgia is a chronic syndrome, it may be necessary over a lengthy period of time to adjust dosages of these medications and/or alternate medications in order to avert dependence or adaptation.

Pain Relief

In severe cases of Fibromyalgia, during a major flare-up, trigger point injections of an analgesic or cortisone medication given directly at the trigger point sites have proven to be helpful in relieving soft tissue pain and breaking up severe muscle spasms.[25]

But for the relentless and constant day-to-day pain there is really very little the medical community can do. Normal pain relievers such as aspirin, acetaminophen, non-steroidal anti-inflammatory drugs (NSAIDS), such as ibuprofen, naproxyn or Aleve or even Cox II inhibitors such as Celebrex, have not proven to be very effective for the pain of Fibromyalgia. Narcotic pain relievers and corticosteroids such as prednisone haven't been shown to be effective for Fibromyalgia pain either.[26]

So what do doctors recommend? Exercise. That's right. Exercise. It sounds all too cruel to tell a person suffering the exhaustion and muscular and joint pains of Fibromyalgia that he or she should exercise.[27] But, believe it or not, the reasoning is sound.

It's because physical exercise releases the body's own natural pain-relieving endorphins.[29] Exercise has been proven to alleviate much of the pain of Fibromyalgia.

Pain management programs recommended by your rheumatologist or local medical facility can be of tremendous help. These pain management groups understand physical pain and work with you. We're not talking Tai Bo or Jumping Jacks here. These are exercises for pain management. Gentle, slow five minute workouts of low or NO-impact stretches are all that's required at first to get those endorphins charged up again.

"Start low and go slow." Add a minute or two each week to your regimen. The relief after each session is truly a blessing.

Note: Recently the FDA has approved a new medication called pregabalin, i.e., Lyrica, to treat Fibromyalgia. Studies show that pregabalin has reduced signs and symptoms of Fibromyalgia in some people.[29] Be aware, however, that since chemical sensitivity is one of the symptoms many FMS sufferers endure, some chemical treatments may not be handled well by a Fibromyalgic body.

If your physician prescribes pregabalin, please be certain to let him or her know immediately if side effects are experienced or if symptoms become worse.

Your health care provider or rheumatologist may also have recommendations as to activities, conditions or foods to avoid. These are called aggravators.

Part II

Aggravators and Options

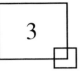

3

Aggravators

Identifying activities, foods, conditions, even *things* that aggravate this syndrome are essential to managing Fibromyalgia. Sufferers must become detectives and find out for themselves what their aggravators are. The list of various and potential aggravators is long and diverse and since space is limited only fifteen of the most common aggravators are listed here, then each is explored in more detail with suggestions for how to minimize each. Some aggravators are as follows:

> Lack of restorative sleep
> Intense pain upon waking
> Lack of exercise
> Too much exercise
> Stress (at home and/or work)
> Hormonal fluctuations (menses or menopause)
> Changes in weather
> Cold and drafty conditions (winter *and* summer air
>   conditioning)
> Erratic daily schedule (at home and/or work)
> Sitting or standing for a lengthy period of time
> Sitting on soft or over-stuffed furniture

Sleeping on a hard or extra firm mattress

Some foods are suspect such as aspartame, sugar, high
fructose corn syrup and nightshades

Extreme ratio of Omega 6 to Omega 3 (essential
fatty acids)

Minimizing these, and any other aggravators the FMS sufferer
may discover in his or her own specific case, is a big step toward
managing Fibromyalgia pain.

Minimizing The Aggravators

1. Lack of restorative sleep. Start with the obvious. Talk to
your doctor. It is helpful, immediately after diagnosis, to hit the
sleep issue with the big guns, with the prescription medications of
Elavil or Flexeril, for example. With normal sleep, which *includes*
the healing Stage 4 sleep, the body can begin to repair itself and
bring in the oxygen it needs on a daily basis. After a couple of
months, when the body is once again familiar with normal sleep,
you may consider switching to a natural supplement like 5HTP
or Melatonin (see **Herbs and Supplements**) and phase off of
the prescriptions.

Prescriptions and supplements aren't the only way to get
sleep, though. You need to do your part. This includes some of
the age-old common sense factors, such as:

—Avoid caffeine and alcohol in the afternoon and evening. This includes soft drinks, chocolate and some medications.

—Avoid spicy foods or drinking water before bed. Heartburn and/or trips to the bathroom don't allow for a peaceful night's sleep.

—On the other hand, a glass of warm milk or a cup of Chamomile tea can be helpful to many.

—Avoid exercising at least three hours before bedtime. Although exercise creates endorphins for helping pain, it is also stimulating and can keep you awake.

—Give yourself time to wind down before bed. Avoid working around the house or on the computer or doing any mentally taxing chores before going to bed.

—Take a soothing bath, listen to relaxing music, read a couple of chapters of a soothing novel (no suspense or horror novels here). Relax your body as well as your mind before going to bed.

—Go to bed at approximately the same time every night. Regularity of schedule is very important. Your body needs to understand that this time of night is for sleep.

—Keep the sleeping room for sleep. A television, computer, telephone, and so on in the bedroom are there to keep you alert. (This includes your cell phone.) A dark, cool, *quiet* atmosphere is much more conducive to sleep.

—Deep breathing exercises, relaxation techniques and visualization exercises are very helpful.

2. Intense pain upon waking.[30] For Fibromyalgia sufferers the hardest part of the day is getting out of bed after lying still for hours at a time. Remaining in one position for any length of time is not in the best interest of a painful Fibromyalgic body.

Upon waking in the morning try this exercise. *Before* you get out of bed, turn to lie on your back. With feet together (as if your big toes were tied together), heels resting on the bed, use your ankles to slowly draw a large circle with your big toes—first clockwise four times, then counterclockwise four times. Rest. Then, scrunch the toes on your left foot as if grabbing something. Hold for a count of four. Relax your toes. Then scrunch the toes on your right foot. Hold for a count of four. Relax your toes. Repeat four times with each foot. Rest. Now point your left foot toward the end of the bed while pointing your right foot toward your forehead. Hold for a count of four. Reverse positions pointing your right foot toward the end of the bed, your left toward your forehead. Repeat four times with each foot. Rest. Now turn on your side for a few minutes (either side will do) and lay in a comfortable fetal position with your pelvis tipped forward, but relaxed. Then slowly, gently get out of bed. The pain will be *much* less severe upon rising.

These exercises get the blood flowing throughout your body. Like starting a car on a cold winter morning; exercising gets the fluids flowing through your engine before putting it in gear.

These toe and ankle exercises are excellent for anyone, with or without Fibromyalgia, who sits at a desk or in a car, on a train or a plane for long periods. They get the blood flowing in the lower extremities and help in breaking up any toxins that settle there over a lengthy period of time.

3. Lack of Exercise. Lack of movement creates pain in a Fibromyalgic body.[31] Exercise, in Fibromyalgic terms, does *not* mean strength training, weight lifting or jogging. Walking from the front of the house to the back of the house can constitute exercise for a person with Fibromyalgia. Walking to the end of the block and back is exercise. Walking up a flight of stairs…you get the idea. This may not seem like much to non-FMS sufferers, but for someone with Fibromyalgia these little trips can be daunting at times. However, they ARE examples of exercise. A person who suffers from Fibromyalgia MUST move, then rest, then move. We will call it exercise for lack of a better term. Do what you can, BUT DO regularly.[32]

When feeling strong enough go to the library and check out VHS tapes (or DVDs) such as *Tai Chi For Arthritis, Stretching for Seniors* (no matter what your age), or similar videos that demonstrate minimal *gentle* exercise. See the suggested list in the chapter on **Resources.**

At home you can try each at your own pace. Just watching the slow, gentle, rhythmic movements of Tai Chi is relaxing and soothing. The benefits of doing these exercises and stretches are a testament unto themselves in the minimizing of Fibromyalgia pain. When you find a video that works well for you, invest in a copy of it for your own personal library. Doing these stretches or exercises with a group is ideal, but doing it with a group on a video is the next best thing in my opinion.

The very best thing about these videos is the ease at which you can pace yourself. You can stop the tape every five minutes if you want, sit down and rest any time you want, and skip over anything you want. You can make up your own exercise regimen using one movement from one tape, two from another and so on. There is no one there to tell you otherwise. Tip: one very important fact of any exercise regimen is to remember what you do on the right side, you must do equally on the left side. This is especially true for a Fibromyalgic body. All four quadrants must get the benefit of the blood and oxygen flowing through those muscles. Balance is the thing.

A regular exercise routine of five minutes a day[33] (or a couple of times a day), then expanding on it next week to six or seven minutes a day and so on, up to fifteen or twenty minutes a day in a month or two, if you can, will bring untold relief from the most severe pain. Remember, "Start low and go slow."

Create a habit for health. Getting into the habit of an exercise regimen can be the very best thing you can do for yourself. You will definitely feel better and you'll find it is extremely meditative and calming. If you're having a painful day, do a two-minute exercise. But do it.

Mornings are ideal for exercising, but early afternoon is good for a pick-me up during a taxing day. As stated earlier, however, don't do these energizing exercises two or three hours before bed as they are not conducive to sleep.

4. Too much exercise. Too much exercise exacerbates Fibromyalgic pain; that's obvious to anyone with Fibromyalgia. But how much is too much? This becomes self-evident when it occurs. Learn your limitations. It's true; these limitations may adjust as these aggravators get more under control, but in the meantime, accept that you simply cannot do what you did before Fibromyalgia. Your body is telling you *change* is needed. Listen to it. Pace yourself realistically for your condition.[34]

5. Stress. It's now common knowledge how much damage stress can do to a body, ranging from ulcers to a heart attack and all kinds of maladies in between, including depression. But illness itself is stressful to a body, especially when it's been three or more months of the exhaustion, pain and confusion of Fibromyalgia. And now it seems that all those little things at home and work, that were never stressful before, have suddenly become disproportionately stressful. They may seem intolerable, even insurmountable.

Those with Fibromyalgia MUST make the time to de-stress.[35] It's as simple as

A, B, C: A is for air, B is for "bye," and C is for count.

A. Learn to breathe. Close your eyes and take deep belly breaths. Breathe in through your nose for a slow count of four. Hold it for a count of four. Then release *all* your breath through pursed lips to a slow count of four. Hold it for a count of four. Repeat as often as you wish. In with the good air, out with the bad.

B. Detach yourself. Physically. Go into the bathroom. Lock the door. Toss a towel onto the floor and take off your socks and shoes. Sit down on the toilet seat and grab the towel with your toes, alternating the right foot and the left. Breathe.

> **Note: When you lock yourself in the bathroom stall at work there may be no towel, so grab your socks with your toes.**

    C. Count. While in the bathroom (or stall) close your eyes and count the big, white, puffy cumulous clouds drifting overhead. In your mind's eye notice their shapes as they drift by, the irregular edges. Feel the puff of wind on your cheek as it pushes the cloud along and the next one drifts into view. Or count M&Ms. Visualize a huge pile of 1,000 M&Ms. Mentally slide one off to the side noticing its color and smooth, round texture as it easily slides over. Listen to the sound it makes as it slides. Mentally pull out another and slide it over, then another and another. Count sheep, or anything having nothing to do with what's on the other side of that locked door.

    The above are called visualization techniques and can be very helpful in calming and de-stressing the body. The toe grips keep the muscles moving (many muscles, if you'll notice); the deep breathing oxygenates the blood and muscles; the visualization calms the stress chemicals. All three help bring the body back into balance. The moving center, the intellectual center and the emotional center all come into balance. Make it a new habit. It will do the body good.

    6. Hormonal fluctuations. Medical assistance may be required here.[36] Dr. Jacob Teitelbaum, best selling author and leading authority on Chronic Fatigue Syndrome uses the acronym

"*SHIN*" to address the treatment of the pain and fatigue of Fibromyalgia. *S* is for sleep, *H* is for hormone balance, *I* is for infection control, and *N* is for nutritional support. "The important thing is that all four should be implemented in concert with one another for maximum therapeutic effect," Dr. Teitelbaum says.

The previously mentioned *locked door* technique may also be helpful.

7. Changes in weather. There's not much one can do about the weather, unfortunately, but the FMS sufferer can prepare for it. Know what's coming and dress appropriately. Err on the side of too much clothing in wet and cold weather. Layers can always be taken off. In winter it helps to wear a hood attached to the coat instead of a hat with a coat. And zip up to your chin. The hood and high neck keep the cold wind off the back of the neck, front of the neck and clavicle areas where trigger points can be affected. Don't get caught without the ability to cover up.

8. Cold and drafty conditions. Don't get caught without the ability to cover up. That is an intentional redundancy. The importance of this cannot be stressed enough. A cold draft to neck, shoulders, arms and hips can cause cramps and pain to increase in intensity. In the summertime be sure to have a long-sleeved shirt handy. Keep one in the car in case it's needed to keep the chill of air conditioning off those sensitive areas.

9. Erratic daily schedule. Home or work schedules that require waking, eating and going to bed at different times every day can play havoc with Fibromyalgia.[35] It is extremely important to wake, exercise, eat, work and go to bed at the same times every day. A regular routine enables the endorphins from exercise and work to be released at regular intervals. Medications and supplements should be taken daily at regular times. Irregular and constantly changing patterns in exercise, work, sleep, etc, prevent the medications, endorphins, the sleep cycle and all the rest from working together efficiently to help ease the pain of Fibromyalgia.

10. Repetitive movements. Computer work, factory work, and even vacuuming require repetitive movements and create pain for a Fibromyalgic body.[37] Shift positions every twenty minutes or so. Do something different; move your body in a different way. If allowed to continually do any one thing for a half hour or more it becomes increasingly difficult to continue that motion. Movement and function may become erratic, not to mention extremely painful.

11. Sitting or standing for a lengthy period of time. Again, shift positions every twenty minutes or so. If sitting, stand and walk around for several minutes. If standing, walk or sit for a several minutes. If walking, sit or stand still for several minutes.[37] Shifting positions every twenty minutes acts like exercise in that the body feels much better *after* the movement. The longer one stays in a single position, the more difficult it is to move into another position. This is one reason the body wakes up in so much pain in the morning.

12. Sitting on soft or overstuffed furniture. This posture bends the body into angles that apply pressure to those sensitive trigger points, especially the neck, shoulders, lower back and hip areas. Ergonomically contoured, molded chairs can also be quite painful to the lower back and hip area. A flat seated, straight backed chair, believe it or not, is really quite comfortable for those with Fibromyalgia. Good posture while sitting or standing keeps pressure off the trigger points, easing pain and aiding function. The very best of all chairs is a flat seated, straight backed rocking chair with or without cushions. This allows the option of movement, always a good thing for a Fibromyalgic body.

13. Sleeping on a hard or extra firm mattress. In the past we've been told that to get a good night's sleep it is necessary to have a good firm mattress. Not so for anyone with Fibromyalgia. A firm mattress can actually apply pressure to some of those very painful trigger points, the lower back and hip areas particularly. Adding a two or three inch foam pad or a pillow top pad to the existing mattress can help reduce this aggravator. Investing in a good air mattress where the softness can be adjusted is quite helpful for some, while one of the popular therapeutic foam mattresses have been helpful for others. Test before you buy. Your health is at stake here.

14. Some foods are suspect.[38] Aspartame (or any chemical sweetener[39]), spicy foods, fried foods, excess sugar (or concentrated sugar, like high fructose corn syrup) and nightshades—a family of foods consisting of tomatoes, white potatoes, green and red bell peppers, hot peppers, eggplant and paprika—have all been shown to aggravate painful symptoms in many people with Fibromyalgia

The best way to find out if aspartame, for example, is an aggravating factor is to eliminate all foods and drinks that contain aspartame for a week to ten days, long enough to flush it out of your system. (Keep in mind that many sugar-free items are sweetened with aspartame; check the labels.) Then begin using those foods and drinks again. If a flare-up occurs in a day or two—sometimes two or three hours will tell—stop using the aspartame again and see if the flare-up subsides. If it does, count aspartame as an aggravator for you. Repeat this test with other chemical sweeteners and foods with high fructose corn syrup.

Do the same with the nightshades, eliminating all for a week to ten days. Then reintroduce them, one each week. Many FMS sufferers will do fine by limiting their diet to one nightshade per meal or per day and never combining two or more at any one meal.

For the past 100 years or so, since processed foods have become our mainstay, Omega 6 fatty acids have been running rampant in our Western diet. From the grocery store to restaurants to fast foods to snack foods, Omega 6 is in practically everything we eat. It is found in vegetable oils from corn, peanut, sesame, safflower, soybean, sunflower, wheat germ and more. It is found in eggs, margarine, poultry, cereals, and baked goods.

In the beginning the Omega 3 in all these products was sufficient to keep these two fatty acids in balance, but Omega 3 fatty acid is obliterated by commercial processing and heat and light, so all that's left of our essential fatty acids, when the food appears on the grocery shelf, is Omega 6.[43] The current high ratio between the two fatty acids (way too much 6 and not enough 3) leads to elevated proinflammatory cytokines, which enhance the risk of other inflammatory diseases such as osteoporosis, arthritis, type 2 diabetes, coronary heart disease, Alzheimer's, and many types of cancer.[41]

Caffeine and carbonated drinks may be an aggravating factor for some. Do the same test with carbonated drinks and coffee. Again, some may do just fine cutting back to one soft drink per day or one or two cups of coffee per day. Also try drinking half water and half coffee, effectively diluting it enough to cause minimal effect.

15. Extreme ratio of Omega 6 to Omega 3. Omega 6 fatty acid has been inadvertently put in the position of being an aggravator. Actually, the inappropriate *ratio* of Omega 6 to Omega 3 has become the aggravator. These essential fatty acids *are* essential and since our body doesn't produce them, we must get them through our diet. The problem is the ratio of the two *should* be 2 or 1:1. But, according to the National Institute of Health (NIH), our Western diet has put it way out of balance at 16 or 20:1, far in favor of Omega 6.[40, 41] (See side bar previous page.)

This excess of Omega-6 fatty acids tends to *increase* inflammation, blood clotting, water retention, cell proliferation, raise blood pressure, have a negative impact on the body's immune system and may contribute to coronary heart disease, arrhythmia, obesity, depression, and some forms of cancer.

Omega 3, on the other hand, when it's brought up in levels to match the intake of Omega 6, *decrease*s inflammation, aids in bringing down blood pressure and blood clotting thereby reducing the risk of cardiovascular disease (CVD), helps regulate arrhythmia, helps relieve water retention, lessen joint pain and bolster the immune system. It has also been shown to help alleviate anxiety, depression and attention deficit disorder. Testing is still being done and more and more benefits are being found when the ratio of Omega 6 and Omega 3 is closer to one-on-one.[42]

There is a little hitch in obtaining this beneficial fatty acid however. Omega 3, containing the all-important EPAs and DHAs, is best obtained through eating dark meat fish like salmon, sardines, swordfish, mackerel and tuna. But eating two or three servings of these fish per week may be prohibitive. Also, according to the FDA, this amount may not be recommended due to possible mercury and PCB content that may be present in these fish.[44]

A good, high quality supplement of Omega 3 fatty acids (Fish Oil), containing the EPA's and DHA's the body needs, seems to be in order here. Fortunately even the best quality Omega 3 supplements, usually from the Netherlands and the North Atlantic Ocean, are not expensive. And since the benefits of Omega 3 have been proven in test
after test, study after study, it is well worth the investment to help alleviate one possible aggravator.[45]

Omega 3 (and Omega 6) is found in walnuts, soy nuts and flaxseed, as well as their oils. But, once again, if the oils are processed or the seeds are heated when used (or the walnuts cooked, as in baked cookies) the Omega 3 is neutralized and you are left with only the Omega 6 fatty acid, adding to an already overabundance of Omega 6 in your body.

Jane Oelke, N.D., Ph.D. describes the role of essential fatty acids as helping to make the cell walls flexible and fluid thereby contributing to the effective transfer of nutrients and oxygen into each cell.

In her book *Natural Choices For Fibromyalgia* Oelke

states, "The one supplement that has made the most difference
[in treating Fibromyalgia] is the use of essential fatty acids in
the diet. If nutrients can't get into the cells the body will never
be healthy."[46]

> (Note: Before taking *any* supplement, check
> with your health care practitioner. Always tell
> your physician of any medications or
> supplements you are currently taking.)

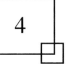

4

Complementary Options

There are many complementary and alternative options for Fibromyalgia sufferers. That said, not all of them work for everyone. And there is no one treatment or combination of treatments that is perfect for every person with Fibromyalgia. But each of the listed therapy treatments below has been shown to help the pain of Fibromyalgia. So each person must decide which treatment or treatments he or she is most comfortable with. This of course means looking into each type of treatment in order to make an informed decision. Most use a combination of several of these therapies.

Acupressure

Acupuncture

Aroma Therapy

Chiropractic Manipulation

Deep -Breathing Exercises

Frequency Specific Microcurrent

Herbs

Hyperbaric Oxygen Therapy

Magnet Therapy

Massage Therapy

Meditation

Myofacial Pain Release Therapy

Nutritional Supplements

Physical Therapy

Pilates

Reflexology

Reiki

Swim/Water Therapy

Tai Chi

Visualization

Walking

Yoga

Most people with Fibromyalgia find a support group extremely helpful. It can be excellent therapy. This can be a group on-line or at a local medical facility, an arthritis support group, a Yoga class, a swim class or what have you. It is comforting to know you are not the only one with this pain. There is the added benefit that others may have found helpful ideas for sleep or pain that may be helpful to you as well.

When looking at the above list, specifically acupressure, chiropractic manipulation, massage therapy, physical therapy, and reflexology, a question may arise.

"Are you crazy? I don't want anyone pushing on me. I hurt when *I* push on me. I hurt when nothing pushes on me."

And the exercise therapies such as Pilates, Tai Chi, Yoga and even walking may seem like they would add pain to an already painful body. But remember those endorphins. These pain-relieving chemicals that are released into your body, with all these touch and movement therapies, work like magic. And remember all the six million or more people with Fibromyalgia who have come before you. They are using these therapies and finding blessed relief. That's where this list came from: other people with Fibromyalgia who recommended them.

Where can you find out about these therapies? All these therapies and more can be found and described in detail on the Internet, of course, but there are more personal and more hands-on means at your disposal. Large cities, medium-size towns and even small towns have libraries, YMCA's, health food stores and hospital facilities.

Acupressure, acupuncture, massage therapy and myofacial pain release therapy are much more available now than ever before and these therapists can usually be found in a telephone book or on a bulletin board or newsletter in a nearby health food store. Hyperbaric oxygen therapy, though not as well known, can usually be found by checking the bulletin board or newsletter at a health food store or by asking the manager or owner of that store. If they don't know of someone practicing the therapy, they can usually find out for you.

A good chiropractor is often found by word of mouth, but they are also listed in the phone book.

Aromatherapy and magnet therapy can be learned through books at the local library or bookstore and of course as stated, the Internet.

Deep breathing exercises, meditation and visualization can be found in books, but consider finding a class through the YMCA, the local health food store or even the library. There's a lot to be said for learning with a small group or class. The good energies are amplified and this may lead to an excellent support group.

Physical therapy is usually found through your rheumatologist or medical health care facility. Swim therapy can be accessed through there, as well as the local YMCA.

The YMCA may also have classes in Yoga, Tai Chi and

Pilates. As mentioned earlier it is also possible to start out slowly by using a video at home.

Reflexology and Reiki healing therapies may be found through the local health food store bulletin board or newsletter, but some medical facilities have listings for these practitioners.

Frequency Specific Microcurrent (FSM) is not yet widely available, but can be found on the Internet. A list of practitioners can be found there as well. This therapy involves an electrical current in the millionth of an ampere (very, very low) and cannot even be felt by the patient.[47] This tiny amount of current can be adjusted to match the exact ampere of the body's own electrical current. It is able to support the natural current flow in tissues, in and around the trigger points and traumatized areas, and helps those painful areas fall back into the patient's proper rhythm. This process helps initiate and perpetuate the many biochemical reactions that occur in healing.[48] FSM therapy seems to have a long lasting effect. Although relatively new, it can certainly be an option for Fibromyalgia pain.

Walking, of course, can be done without any fee or special equipment other than good walking shoes, which is standard for anyone with Fibromyalgia, along with loose, comfortable clothing. It can be done literally anywhere outside, or inside a mall in bad weather.

Herbs and supplements. These may well be among the most helpful treatments for Fibromyalgia pain and restful sleep.

Some of the herbs and supplements recommended by medical doctors, naturopaths, alternative healers, researchers and Fibromyalgia sufferers themselves are: Omega 3, magnesium, malic acid, CoQ10, Eleuthero, Sam-e, garlic extract or olive leaf extract, 5HTP or melatonin, a good high quality multi-vitamin and water.[49, 50]

(Note: Before taking *any* supplement, check with your health care practitioner. Always tell your physician of any medications or supplements you are currently taking.)

Omega 3. Although the body needs both Omega 3 and Omega 6 we clearly have more than enough Omega 6 (inflammatory) fatty acids to sustain us. And just as clearly we need to add Omega 3 to bring back the proper balance. This will help ease pain, lower blood pressure, balance mood, bolster the immune system and more.

Magnesium. Magnesium deficiency is not common. But dietary levels of magnesium in most people are often low, and specific medical conditions can deplete this mineral even more, including prolonged stress. Excess coffee, soft drinks, and alcohol are other depleting factors. Some symptoms of magnesium deficiency are muscle aches and weakness, fatigue, sleepiness, abnormal heart rate, insomnia, anxiety, poor memory and confusion.[51] Magnesium is often teamed with malic acid for pain relief.

Malic acid. Malate is a naturally occurring compound in the body that plays an important role in the production of energy. The supplement of malic acid is an "acid" derived from fruit, mostly apples, which helps the body to make energy even under low oxygen conditions. Along with helping to raise energy levels and ease pain, malic acid also helps remove excessively high levels of phosphorous and aluminum in the body. It is an excellent pain reliever on its own, but even more powerful when teamed with magnesium.[52]

CoQ10. This supplement helps increase the energy level in the body. CoQ10 is found in the mitochondria of each cell in the body and is a natural energy producer involved in a wide range of body systems.[53] This natural enzyme is abundant in infancy but decreases as we age. Since CoQ10 is not water soluble, it must be taken with an oil in order to be absorbed properly. Some brands of this enzyme include a small amount of Vitamin E to aid in its absorption.

Eleuthero (formerly known as Siberian Ginseng). This is an adaptogenic herb that helps the body to adapt to various kinds of stress such as heat, cold, exertion and sleep privation. It is helpful in promoting energy and aids in supporting the immune system.[54]

Sam-e. Sam-e, short for S-adenosylmethionine, is present in every living cell in the body and is involved in many biochemical processes. Sam-e is not found in food; it is produced by the body. However, as we age, the levels of Sam-e tend to decline. This supplement has been shown to improve the pain, fatigue, mood and morning stiffness of Fibromyalgia. In Europe, it is classified as an antidepressant and is a prescription medication used to treat depression, Chronic Fatigue Syndrome, Fibromyalgia, Osteo-arthritis, and more. In the United States it is sold over the counter. Sam-e is not meant to be used with other antidepressant medications, nor should it to be used by people with bi-polar disorder.[55]

Garlic Extract [56, 57] or Olive Leaf Extract.[62] Both provide potent immune system support and powerful antioxidant support. Both help fight off bacteria, viruses and fungus, which is a must for FMS sufferers, since a simple infection or a cold can amplify all the symptoms of Fibromyalgia. Garlic Extract and Olive Leaf Extract may have the added benefit of helping to maintain a healthy heart and circulatory system. Both raise the HDL (good cholesterol) levels and decrease LDL (bad cholesterol) levels, and both are known to lower blood pressure and act as blood thinners. Neither should be used prior to surgery or if Warfarin has been prescribed.

5-HTP or Melatonin. The amino acid 5-hydroxytryptophan (5-HTP) helps the body produce seratonin. It has been shown to improve sleep quality and reduce pain, stiffness, anxiety and depression in Fibromyalgia sufferers.[58]

Melatonin is a hormone secreted by the pineal gland that regulates the biological rhythms associated with light and dark- the circadian rhythm. In other words, it governs the sleep cycle.

Melatonin is helpful for people with jetlag or night workers who have a mixed up day/night schedule.[59]

Ask your health care provider if either of these supplements would be right for you. Neither Melatonin nor 5-HTP should be taken with an antidepressant, a seratonin reuptake inhibitor (SSRI) or a monoamine oxidase inhibitor (MAOI).

Multi-Vitamin. A good, high quality multi-vitamin can help tremendously. This will ensure that your body gets the all important B vitamins and folic acid along with the selenium, niacin, biotin, zinc and all the other essential vitamins that are so crucial for a painful body. The modern western diet is sorely lacking in the most basic of essential nutrients simply due to so much processing and *quick meals,* frozen and otherwise. Give yourself the edge needed to rebuild your most basic resources.

Water. Water is especially important if you are taking supplements, herbs or medications, or if you are retaining fluids. Water enables the supplements to flow into your blood stream and be moved along throughout your muscles and other tissues, delivering their payload. Water helps eliminate acid wastes that build up in a chronically ill body. And if you are retaining fluids, it is important to flush out the old, stale, possibly toxic fluids that are being held in your tissues. Only water counts. Coffee and soft drinks are actually diuretics, causing you to lose water.

How much water? At least 8 full, 8oz glasses of water per day is usually recommended. But Jane Oelke, N.D., PhD. recommends drinking "one-half your weight in ounces of water.

So...if you weigh 150 lbs. you would need 75 ounces of water per day. Spreading out the amount of water throughout the day is easier on the kidneys..."[60]

The point is that water serves a purpose in the body- it is, in fact, quite necessary for the body to function properly. Coffee, soft drinks and alcohol may impair some of those functions, especially when used in excess.

* * *

Fibromyalgia is not a one-treatment-fits-all kind of syndrome. Arm yourself with information. Then get moving...literally. Bit by bit build up your strength, five minutes at a time. See your doctor or rheumatologist; go to your local health food store; go to the library; check out your local YMCA and buy a swimsuit. Join a support group. Sign up for a newsletter to get the latest information on any one of the Fibromyalgia websites. You must be the biggest part of your treatment.

PART III

What to do for you

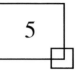

5

Help Yourself

Helping yourself is the very best thing you can do. By seeing your health care provider, avoiding your own particular aggravators and looking into complementary and alternative options, you can be in control of your own health and well-being.

In point of fact, you are the *only* one who can effectively treat your Fibromyalgia, although you may need to brush up on your self-management skills by learning some new skills. Relaxation and deep breathing exercises, maintaining a regular daily schedule, pacing yourself and knowing your limitations are all part of it.

Learn what works for you. Maybe massage therapy, acupuncture, or swim therapy will appeal to you. Walking, Tai Chi, or Pilates may be your cup of tea. Often your own body in the form of a "gut feeling" will tell you what you need to do. Read up on the list of supplements and choose which ones you believe may help you. Your body is not the enemy here. It's simply telling you change is needed. Listen to it.

Dr. D.A. Williams and Dr. M. Carey of the University of Michigan Health System share the most valuable tip of all:

"Pain is associated with negative emotions such as sadness, frustration, and irritability. When people are in pain and also have these emotions, the pain becomes worse. That is because these emotions are processed in the same area of the brain as is pain.

"Research has shown that pain decreases when people experience more positive emotions."[61]

So do something that brings you joy. Go fly a kite. Go fishing. Skip a stone on a pond. Take a walk in the park and watch a squirrel run up a tree. Go out and buy the most huggable stuffed animal you can find. Read a good heart-warming book. Watch an uplifting movie. Work with your hands- do a craft or work a puzzle. Play with your pet. Wear colorful clothes. Bring some light and color into your workplace and your home- bring in some upbeat music while you're at it. Learn to dance. Learn Tai Chi. Smile. Treat yourself to a manicure…a pedicure or a new hairstyle…a massage. Cultivate your sense of humor. Read a joke book. Go out and play in your garden. Start a window garden. Start a journal.

LIFT YOUR LIFE and heal the pain.

Depending on which website you consult there are 3-6 million, 7 million, 10 million, 12 million or 2-4% of the American population who have Fibromyalgia. With the numbers growing at this rate of speed, more and more researchers are hard at work looking for a cure. But maybe a *cure* isn't necessarily what's needed. Maybe it's change that's needed. Change of our lifestyle, our eating habits, our outlook or our ability to be at peace with our body…and those bodies around us.

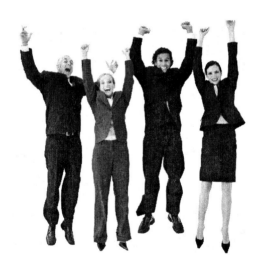

Resources

There are a multitude of resources available for finding out more about Fibromyalgia and how to manage it, as well as finding out about the newest and latest research. Some of them are: your local library, health food store, health care facility, websites, magazines such as "Arthritis Today" and others, your local YMCA and even the phone book under "Physical Therapists," "Pain Management," or "Physicians-Arthritis" to name a few. The sites listed below, books and videos, are a few places to start.

<u>Medical Facilities and their websites</u>:

Arthritis Foundation
http://www.arthritis.org, keyword search- type Fibromyalgia

National Institute of Health Bethesda, MD
National Institute of Arthritis and Musculoskeletal and Skin Diseases (NIAMS)
http://www.niams.nih.gov, click on "F," then Fibromyalgia

Mayo Clinic
Rochester, MN 55905
http://www.mayoclinic.com, type Fibromyalgia, click on "search"

University of Maryland Medical Center
Baltimore, MD 21201
http://www.umm.edu, type Fibromyalgia, click on "go"
http://www.umm.edu/altmed, type Fibromyalgia, click "search"

University of Michigan Health System/Chronic Pain and Fatigue Research Center Ann Arbor, Michigan

> http://www.med.umich.edu/painresearch/patients/
index.htm.
> Click on "Learn about Fibromyalgia"

Healthy Websites:

Health World
> http://www.healthy.net, under "Health Conditions"
> click on Fibromyalgia

Web MD
> http://www.WebMD.com, type Fibromyalgia, click "search"

Fibromyalgia websites:

CFS and Fibromyalgia Solutions For Patients
> http://www.endfatigue.com

Fibromyalgia & Fatigue Centers, Inc.
> http://www.fibroandfatigue,com

Fibromyalgia Network
> http://www.fmnetnews.com

Fibromyalgia-Symptoms
> http://www.fibromyalgia-symptoms.org

National Fibromyalgia Association
> http://www.fmaware.org and www.fibrohope.org

National Fibromyalgia Research Association
  www.nfra.net
Pro Health
  http://www.immunesupport.com

Frequency Specific websites:

Frequency Specific Microcurrent
  http://www.frequencyspecific.com.
  Find a practitioner in your area.

Frequency Specific Microcurrent
  http://pages.prodigy.net/naturedoctor/microcurrent.html.

RiverHill Wellness Center
  http://www.riverhillwellness.com/fibromyalgia.htm.
  Click on "Frequency Specific Microcurrent."

WikipediaThis is an excellent source for hyperlinks to more information.
  http://www.wikipedia.org
  Type "Fibromyalgia," chose your favorite language, and click on the arrow.

Books:

Alternative treatments for Fibromyalgia and Chronic Fatigue Syndrome Second Edition, 2006, by Walker, Mari Skelly and Helen.

The Everything Health Guide to Fibromyalgia 2006, by McNett, Winnie Yu and Michael M. Yu, M.D.

Fibromyalgia & Chronic Myofacial Pain Syndrome: A Survival Manual 1996, By Starlanyl, Devin, M.D. and Copeland, Mary Ellen, M.S., M.A.

Natural Choices For Fibromyalgia 2001
by Oelke, Jane, N.D., Ph.D.

Videos:

Gentle Tai Chi from Terra Entertainment (in a seated position)

Moving To Mozart with Ann Smith

*Stretching For Senior*s with Ann Smith

Tai Chi For Arthritis with Paul Lam

Tai Chi For Back Pain with Paul Lam

Tai Chi For Beginners with Paul Lam

About the Author

Pati Chandler suffered with Fibromyalgia for ten years. During that time she learned a few little "tricks of the trade" that enabled her to juggle working, writing and managing Fibromyalgia all at the same time.

She suffered a multitude of symptoms for about six months before being diagnosed. Pati thought she would never be able to write again. She couldn't sit long enough and couldn't focus.

"I didn't care enough about anything except how much I hurt. I thought I'd never work again."

Chandler just knew she would be in a wheel chair soon and wouldn't even be able to get into her home.

"Depressed? You bet. My life changed absolutely."

Chandler tells us she's a "researchaholic." Once she was diagnosed, she *had* to find out all about the *syndrome* that wasn't considered serious enough to be called a disease. Ten years ago there was precious little out there to be found, but she "ate up" what she did find.

Although Pati Chandler has no medical credentials, she has been doing her own research on Fibromyalgia since day one, the day she learned the name of all the symptoms she was experiencing.

She remembers that day well....

"I remember that day well. I hadn't been to a doctor for years and I was afraid he was going to lock me up and throw away the key when he heard all my symptoms and complaints. Thus I decided to tell him only a few."

She claims not having a family doctor back then and figured if he thought she was crazy, she would never have to see him again.

"I had visions of being in a wheel chair with MS or in a nursing home for 52-year-olds with Alzheimer's." She confesses to being there out of desperation, wanting desperately to get rid of her pain.

After describing the pain Chandler had been experiencing for the prior six months, her doctor finally asked her how she felt upon waking in the morning.

"When I told him, he gently laid his finger on my skin near my clavicle. The pain he evoked brought me to tears as I pulled away from him."

Doc raised his eyebrows, nodded his head and said, "Uh-huh."

"Through my tears and pain I said, 'What uh-huh?'"

The doctor somehow convinced her to sit there while he proceeded to lay his finger on seventeen more pressure points. When he finished, she was in severe pain everywhere and wet from sweating as if she had just stepped from a swimming pool. He mentioned the word *Fibromyalgia,* but Chandler was too out-of-it at the time to respond even with a question mark, she said.

"I sat and cried with pain as he left the room."

When her doctor returned, he had written down the names of a couple of websites, and a book, telling Pati that some doctors think Fibromyalgia is a myth, or it is actually myofacial pain syndrome with a twist, or that's it all in her head. That's because there is no proof it exists, medically speaking.

Great, she thought. She had a non-existent *syndrome* with a weird name. "So how do you fix it?" Chandler asked.

He shook his head and wrote her a prescription for Elavil.

About two months later she was feeling a bit better, at least was sleeping better. But then she woke up one morning and discovered she couldn't turn her head. The doctor gave her trigger point injections in the back of her neck and shoulder area. In a few days Pati was instructed to start doing gentle neck and shoulder exercises as a follow-up to these injections, and to ensure those muscles didn't freeze up again. She says she still does them, and more.

"I thank God every day that this relatively young doctor knew his stuff."

Back in 1998, Fibromyalgia was not a common syndrome, much less a common word. The author began her research on-line that same day. She could only sit for fifteen minutes at a time and it was slow going, but the bits and pieces she assembled confirmed what her doctor revealed. Many doctors did not *believe* in Fibromyalgia. But Chandler persisted. This book is the result of her accumulated outstanding research.

"Throughout the course of these ten years my life has changed drastically."

Ms. Chandler said she gave up her dream job of nine years with the Department of Natural Resources. She could no longer work outside in the winter. She now works part-time indoors at a large retail store. She changes her shoes three times a day because what is comfortable in the morning is no longer comfortable at noon. Still, she wears only good supportive shoes.

"I couldn't sit in my new Lazy-Boy, so I got a secondhand bentwood rocker, which is now *my chair*. I couldn't sit in my car for more than a few minutes without experiencing severe pain, so I had the car seat re-upholstered." She wears sunglasses year 'round; has two pair in the car, plus a pair in her purse.

"I never used to take pills," she says, "not even aspirin. Now I take up to 7 supplements three times a day. I was never a breakfast person, but I did to learn to eat in the morning because I need the energy and my supplements are best taken with food."

She no longer drinks carbonated soft drinks. Instead, she eats a lot more whole, fresh foods than ever before, comsumes much less sugar and fewer sweets.

"I really learned to love fresh veggies. Who would have guessed?"

Chandler bought a rubber cone-shaped gizmo so she could open jars and milk containers, due to having no grip in her hands. She keeps scissors in every room to open everything…from a bag of cereal to a new cellophane-wrapped magazine to a card of roller ball pens. She buys the large bodied pens, which are easier to hold.

After admitting to being a former drinker of coffee by the potful, Ms. Chandler now drinks only two cups of coffee a day and they are both half hot water and half coffee. She also drinks lots of water and green tea. She claims that before Fibromyalgia this would never have happened.

Ms. Chandler asks the grocery bag person to fill her canvas bags lightly and, as a result, makes more trips bringing them into the house. She keeps everything in its proper place so when fibro-fog hits, she can still find it. "Almost," she clarifies. "I always keep gloves handy so I can hold a cold glass of water or take frozen food out of the freezer.

"I do the dishes in two stages, sitting to rest periodically. I change the bed sheets, vacuum and do laundry the same way, of course. I bought a sleep number bed (I am a number 40). I do toe and ankle exercises before I get out of bed. I meditate and do Tai Chi exercises every morning and sometimes in the afternoon."

Chandler avoids going out after nine p.m. Instead, she uses the hour before her ten o'clock bedtime to wind down and relax. She does not attend large public events where the noise would be intolerable. She carries earplugs in her purse anyway, because she never knows when she'll go to a movie with the grandkids.

"Of course, I have a flannel shirt in the car in case it's cold in the movie theater. Planning ahead is always a good idea."

Another thing Chandler always carries in her purse is a box of mints. It's her first-aid kit to nausea and flatulence. "Peppermint oil (not simply mint-flavor, but the oil) is a must to have on hand. Thank you, Junior Mints™."

She bought a painter's facemask to cover her nose and mouth when her husband is painting or working in the basement with paint thinners, glues and such.

"I always have a fleece jacket or fleece wrap nearby, even in the summer, to keep chills off my neck and shoulders, hips and knees." Among her essentials she bought a winter coat that zips up over her chin and has a hood to keep the wind chill off those nasty trigger points. In addition, she buys only loose-fitting, comfortable clothing. Chandler learned early on about the negative effects of tight jeans and turtlenecks.

"I try to stay upbeat. Fortunately I still have my sense of humor. I wear light-colored clothes, watch uplifting or funny movies and listen to soothing or light tempo music. I play with my cats, read lighthearted, romantic mystery novels, surround myself with light-colored walls, brightly colored accents and the things I enjoy. I have learned to LIFT my LIFE."

These are a few of Pati Chandler's life adaptations to Fibromyalgia. But she is now able to sit at her computer, while exercising her feet and ankles regularly (long enough to research and write this booklet). Fibromyalgia is still with her. But by using a few little tricks described here: supplements, meditation, deep breathing exercises, Tai Chi exercises, and avoiding her aggravators, she has learned to manage her Fibromyalgia.

"I still have a bad day now and then, but doesn't everyone? "If I can help even one other soul learn to manage her or his Fibromyalgia symptoms, then I consider my mission accomplished. I thank God for the opportunity to do so."

Ms. Chandler knows Fibromyalgia will change your life. That is a given. But you can choose what direction that change will take. Lifestyle adaptations may very well be necessary. For some, this may mean a change in the workplace or even a change of job entirely. New concepts like Frequency Specific Microcurrent, and old concepts like Tai Chi, are here now. New methodologies and old-fashioned supplements like fish oil are here now.

"Fellow sufferer, you are in charge of the rest of your life. Choose to help yourself."

Biography

Pati Chandler lives in Mishawaka, Indiana, with her husband and four cats. She is the mother of four children and grandmother of six.

A diverse background of studies at the University of Indiana at South Bend in the 1980's included many classes in psychology, criminal justice, philosophy and journalism earning her an Associates Degree in General Studies.

From security work at the University, then at the security checkpoint at the local airport, she moved on to her real love working for the Department of Natural Resources (DNR). In 1998, after nine years with the DNR, she contracted Fibromyalgia and was forced to leave her job and focus on her health. She now works thirty hours a week at a large retail department store.

She enjoys reading and watching movies that leave a smile on her face. She is a tree-hugger and animal lover, finding the joy and beauty in nature an inspiration for her writing.

Endnotes

[1] WebMD. Fibromyalgia Guide. *Understanding Fibromyalgia-the Basics. Who is Affected?* 2007. http://www.webmd.com/fibromyalgia/guide/understanding-fibromyalgia-basics.

[2] National Institute of Arthritis and Musculoskeletal and Skin Disease (NIAMS). *Questions and Answers About Fibromyalgia.* 1999. http://www.niams.nih.gov/Health_Info/Fibromyalgia/default.asp. Para 2.

[3] MayoClinic.com. *Fibromyalgia- Introduction.* 2007. http://www.mayoclinic.com/health/fibromyalgia/DS00079. Para 2.

[4] University of Michigan Health System (UMHS). Health Topics A-Z. *Fibromyalgia- What is Fibromyalgia?* 2007. http://www.med.umich.edu/1libr/aha/umfibromyalgia.htm.

[5] MayoClinic.com. *Fibromyalgia- Signs and Symptom- Other common signs and symptoms include.* 2007. http://www.mayoclinic.com/health/fibromyalgia/DS00079/DSECTION=2.

[6] American Chronic Pain Association. *Biography of founder Penney Cowan.* http://theacpa.org/nerve/bios.asp. Para 4.

[7] UMHS. Chronic Pain and Fatigue Research Center. *For Health Care Provides- Diagnosis.* 1996. http://www.med.umich.edu/painresearch/pro/diagnosis.htm. Para 3.

[8] MayoClinic.com. *Fibromyalgia- Signs & Symptoms.* 2007.
http://www.mayoclinic.com/health/fibromyalgia/DS00079/
DSECTION=2.

[9] MayoClinic.com. *Fibromyalgia- When to seek medical
advice.* 2007. http://www.mayoclinic.com/health/fibromyalgia/
DS00079/DSECTION=5.

[10] Wellness.com. Condition by Name. *Fibromyalgia- What
causes it?* 2006.
http://www.wellness.com/conditions.asp?RequestUrl=/resources/
Complementary%20and%20Alternative%20Medicine/
33_Condition_idx.htm. Para 4.

[11] UMHS. Chronic Pain and Fatigue Research Center. *For
Patients- Self-Management Skills & Techniques- Sleep.*
Williams, D.A. and Carey, M. *You Really Need To Sleep.* 2003.
http://www.med.umich.edu/painresearch/patients/sleep.pdf.
Page 1.

[12] National Fibromyalgia Association (NFA). *Fibromyalgia.
What are the symptoms? Pain.* http://www.fmaware.org/site/
PageServer?pagename=fibromyalgia_symptoms.

[13] Starlanyl and Copeland. *Fibromyalgia & Chronic Myofacial
Pain Syndrome.* 1996. CA, New Harbringer Publications, Inc.
p127.

[14] Fibromyalgia & Fatigue Centers, Inc. *About Fibromyalgia.*
http://fibroandfatigue.com/aboutfibromyalgia.php. Para 6.

[15] University of Maryland Medical Center (UMM). *Medical
reference-Encyclopedia. Fibromyalgia-Overview-Causes,
incidence and risk factors.* 2006. http://www.umm.edu/ency/
article/000427.htm. Para 2.

[16] NIAMS. *Questions and Answers About Fibromyalgia-What Causes Fibromyalgia?* 1999. http://www.niams.nih.gov/Health_Info/Fibromyalgia/default.asp.

[17] NFA. *Fibromyalgia. What Causes Fibromyalgia?* http://www.fmaware.org/site PageServer?pagename=fibromyalgia_causes.

[18] MayoClinic.com. *Fibromyalgia- Screening and Diagnosis.* 2007. http://www.mayoclinic.com/health/fibromyalgia/DS00079/Dsection=6

[19] UMHS. Chronic Pain and Fatigue Research Center. *For Patients- Fibromyalgia-Diagnosis-The criteria include.* 1996. http://www.med.umich.edu/painresearch/pro/fibromyalgia.htm

[20] UMM. *Altmed-Articles-Fibromyalgia.* 2006. http://www.umm.edu/altmed/articles/fibromyalgia-000061.htm

[21] UMHS. Arthritis & Rheumatism. Gracely, R.H., Petzke, F, Wolf, J.M., Clauw, D.J. 2002. *Functional Magnetic Resonance Imaging Evidence of Augmented Pain Processing in Fibromyalgia.* http://www.med.umich.edu/opm/newspage/2002/clauw%20paper.pdf

[22] WebMD. Fibromyalgia Guide. *Overview & Facts-Fibromyalgia- Causes.* 2007. http://www.webmd.com/fibromyalgia/guide/fibromyalgia-causes

[23] MayoClinic.com. *Fibromyalgia. Treatment- medications-antidepressants.* 2007. http://www.mayoclinic.com/health/fibromyalgia/DS00079/DSECTION=8

[24] UMM. *Altmed-Articles-S-adenosylmethionine-overview.* 2002.
http://www.umm.edu/altmed/articles/s-adenosylmethionine-000324.htm. Para 2.

[25] UMM. *Altmed-Articles-Fibromyalgia. Treatment Options-drug therapies.* 2006. http://www.umm.edu/altmed/articles/fibromyalgia-000061.htm. Para 5.

[26]MayoClinic.com. *Fibromyalgia. Treatment- medications.* 2007. http://www.mayoclinic.com/health/fibromyalgia/DS00079/DSECTION=8. Para 10.

[27] American College of Rheumatology. *Patient education. Fibromyalgia- Living with Fibromyalgia.* 2006. http:/www.rheumatology.orgpublicfactsheetsfibromya_new.asp?#6. Para 4.

[28] MayoClinic.com. *Exercise takes the edge off chronic pain-The benefits of movement.* 2007. http://www.mayoclinic.com/health/chronic-pain/AR00017. Para 2.

[29] MayoClinic.com. *Fibromyalgia- Treatment-medications-pregabalin.* 2007. http://www.mayoclinic.com/health/fibromyalgia/DS00079/DSECTION=8.

[30] National Fibromyalgia Partnership. *FM Monograph- Other conditions Associated with FM- stiffness.* 2006. http://www.fmpartnership.org/Files/Website2005/Learn%20About%20Fibromyalgia/FM%20Overview/Monograph—English.htm

[31] MayoClinic.com. *Exercise takes the edge off chronic pain-The risks of inactivity.* 2007. http://www.mayoclinic.com/health/chronic-pain/AR00017.

65

32 UMHS. Health Topics A-Z. *Fibromyalgia- How is it treated?* 2007. http://www.med.umich.edu/1libr/aha/ umfibromyalgia.htm. Para 4.

33 UMHS. Chronic Pain and Fatigue Research Center. *For Health Care Providers- Non-pharmacologic Therapies.* http://www.med.umich.edu/painresearch/pro/fm-nonpharm.htm.

34 UMHS. Chronic Pain and Fatigue Research Center. *For Patients- Self-Management Skills & Techniques-Pacing.* Williams, D.A. and Carey, M. *Improve Your Functioning Through Effective Pacing.* 2003. http://www.med.umich.edu/painresearch/patients/pacing.pdf. Page 3.

35 UMHS. Health Topics A-Z. *Fibromyalgia- How is it treated?* 2007. http://www.med.umich.edu/1libr/aha/umfibromyalgia.htm. Para 6.

36 Healthy.Net. Teitelbaum, Jacob, MD. *Pain Free 1-2-3! A Proven Program to Get Patients Pain-Free.* http://www.healthy.net/scr/column.asp?Id=624. Para 3.

37 NFA. *An Overview for the Newly Diagnosed Patient. The Treatment of Fibromyalgia.* http://www.fmaware.org/site/ PageServer?pagename=fibromyalgia_overview. Para 7

38 WebMD. Fibromyalgia Guide. *Early Symptoms of Fibromyalgia- What are the symptoms?* http://www.webmd.com/fibromyalgia/guide/understanding-fibromyalgia-symptoms. Item 9.

66

[39] Oelke, J. MI, Natural Choices, Inc. *Natural Choices For Fibromyalgia* 2001 Pp130-131

[40,] NIH. National Center for Biotechnology. *Pubmed- The importance of the ratio of omega-6/omega essential fatty acids. The Center for Genetics, Nutrition and Health, Washington, D.C.20009 USA.* 2002.
http://www.ncbi.nlm.nih.gov/pubmed/12442909.

[41,] UMM. *Altmed- articles-Omega-3 fatty acids- overview.* 2007. http://www.umm.edu/altmed/articles/omega-3-000316.htm.
Para 3.

[42] NIH. Office of Dietary Supplements. *Omega 3 Fatty Acids and Health. Background information about omega-3 and omega-6 fatty acids and their unknown functions.* 2005.
http://www.ods.od.nih.gov/FactSheets/
Omega3FattyAcidsandHealth_pf.asp. Para 4.

[43] University of Cincinnati, Ohio State University. *Health Topics-Complementary Medicine- Understanding Omega-3 and Omega-6.* 2005.
http://www.netwellness.org/healthtopics/alternative/
Omega3.cfm. Para 2.

[44] U.S. Food and Drug Administration (FDA). *Mercury In Fish:Cause For Concern?* 1994.
http://www.fda.gov/fdac/reprints/mercury.html.

[45] UMM. *Altmed- articles- Omega 3- Uses.* 2007.
http://www.umm.edu/altmed/articles/omega-3-000316.htm

[46] Oelke, J. MI: Natural Choices, Inc. *Natural Choices for Fibromyalgia.* 2001. Pp107-110.

[47] Lee, J.M. Naturopathic Physician. *Treatment Modalities-Commonly Asked Questions About Frequency Specific Microcurrent.* http://www.leenaturopathic.com/microcurrent.htm. Para 4.

[48] Frequency Specific Microcurrent. *Welcome to Frequency Specific Microcurrent.* 2007. http://www.frequencyspecific.com

[49.] UMM. *Altmed- articles-Fibromyalgia-Treatment Options-Nutrition and Supplements.* 2006. http://www.umm.edu/altmed/articles/fibromyalgia-000061.htm

[50] Wellness.com. Conditions by Name. *Fibromyalgia-Complementary and Alternative Therapies-Nutrition and Supplements.* 2006. http://www.wellness.com/conditions.asp?RequestUrl=/resources/Complementary%20and%20Alternative%20Medicine/33_Condition_idx.htm

[51] UMM. *Altmed-articles-Magnesium- Overview.* http://www.umm.edu/altmed/articles/magnesium-000313.htm. Para 3

[52] Healing With Nutrition. *Missing Nutrients Linked to Fibromyalgia and Chronic Pain- Missing Nutrients.* 2001. http://www.healingwithnutrition.com/fdisease/fibromyalgia/magnesiumstudy.html. Para 3.

[53] UMM. *Altmed-articles-CoQ10- Overview.* http://www.umm.edu/altmed/articles/coenzyme-q10-000295.htm

68

[54] UMM. *Altmed-articles-Siberian ginseng- Overview.*
http://www.umm.edu/altmed/articles/siberian-ginseng-
000250.htm. Para 2.

[55] UMM. *Altmed-articles-Sam-e- Precautions.*
http://www.umm.edu/altmed/articles/s-adenosylmethionine-
000324.htm. Para 3.

[56] UMM. *Altmed-articles-Garlic-Overview.*
http://www.umm.edu/altmed/articles/garlic-000245.htm

[57] American Academy of Anti-Aging Medicine. *Anti-Aging
Library. Botanical Agents- Olive Leaf Extract.*
http://www.worldhealth.net/p/aadr-olive-leaf-extract-olea-
europa.html.

[58] UMM. *Altmed-articles- 5-HTP- Overview.*
http://www.umm.edu/altmed/articles/5-htp-000283.htm

[59] UMM. *Altmed- articles-Melatonin- Overview.*
http://www.umm.edu/altmed/articles/melatonin-000315.htm

[60] Oelke, J., 2001 MI, Natural Choices, Inc. *Natural Choices for
Fibromyalgia.* 2001. Pp123-125.

[61] UMHS. Chronic Pain and Fatigue Research Center. *For
Patients. Self-Management Skills & Techniques-Pacing.*
Williams, D.A. and Carey, M. *Improve Your Functioning
Through Effective Pacing.* 2003.
http://www.med.umich.edu/painresearch/patients/pacing.pdf.
Page 8.

MAIL-IN REORDER FORM

Customer Name (Please print legibly)

Street Address _____ **Apt** _____

City   **State**   **Zip**

P.O. Box _____   Note: If you have a street address
and PO box you must include both
on this form if paying by credit card.

Phone: (   ) _____

Order Qty $14.95 $8.00

                 [   ]   [   ]

                 Hardback   Paperback

                                              <u>Amount Paid</u>

Payment by Check

(Enclosed) _____ $ _____

                              Arizona Residents
                              Add 7.85% Sales Tax _____

                              Shipping/Handling _____

Payment by Visa
MasterCard or Discover   **Total** $ _____

Card No. _____

Expiration Date: _____

CVV Code
(last three digits) _____

Web site http://www.trebleheartbooks.com